DELICIOUS VEGETARIAN DISHES
THE 10 BEST RECIPES

Dana Priyanka Hammond

Contents

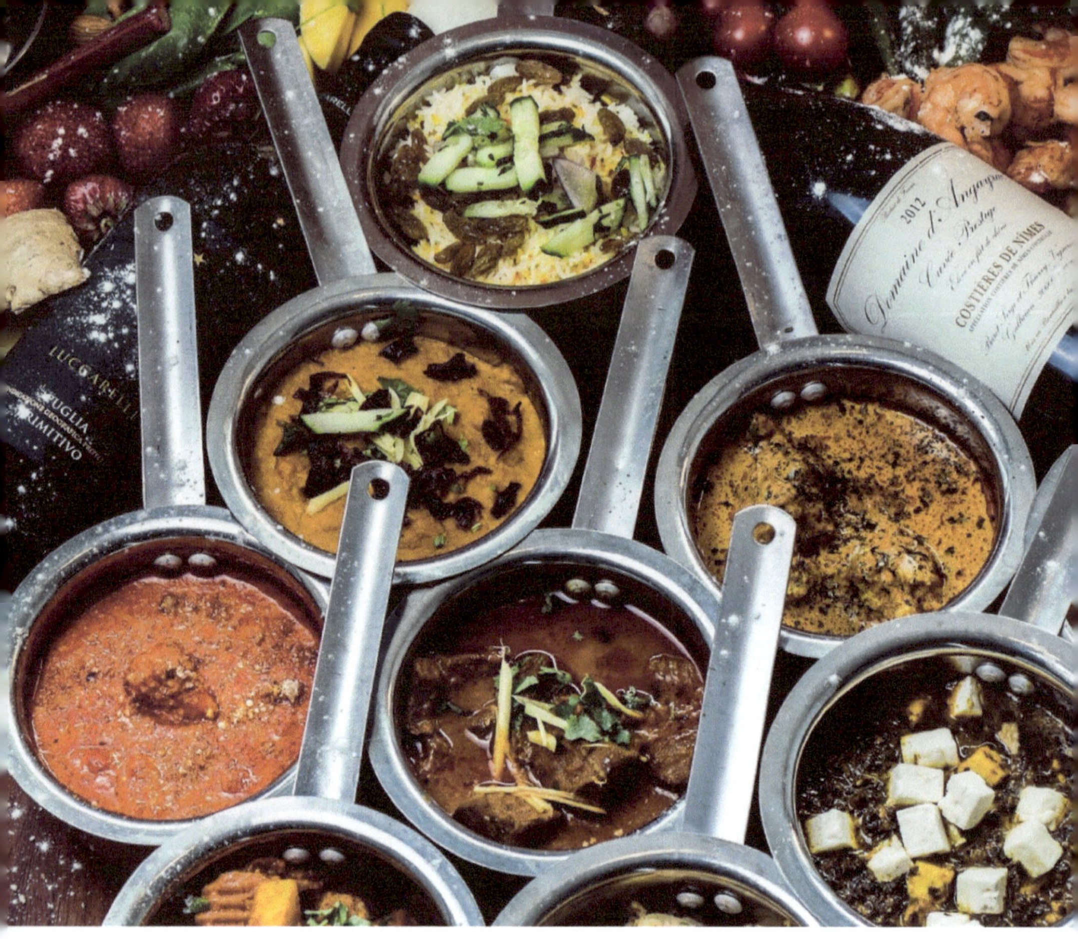

ACKNOWLEDGEMENT

I dedicate this book to my friend Julie Knight. Julie has been my biggest encouragement in believing to knowing that all things are possible and that it is time to let my wings expand. Thank you for your motivation and inspiration... She has inspired me to do well even in my cooking and to better myself. When the opportunity prevailed to follow my dreams, I never imagined that I would have an opportunity to create a cookbook. Her dedication and prayers to cover me as I pursued this dream has been heard by God who grants me an opportunity to write an Indian Cookbook.

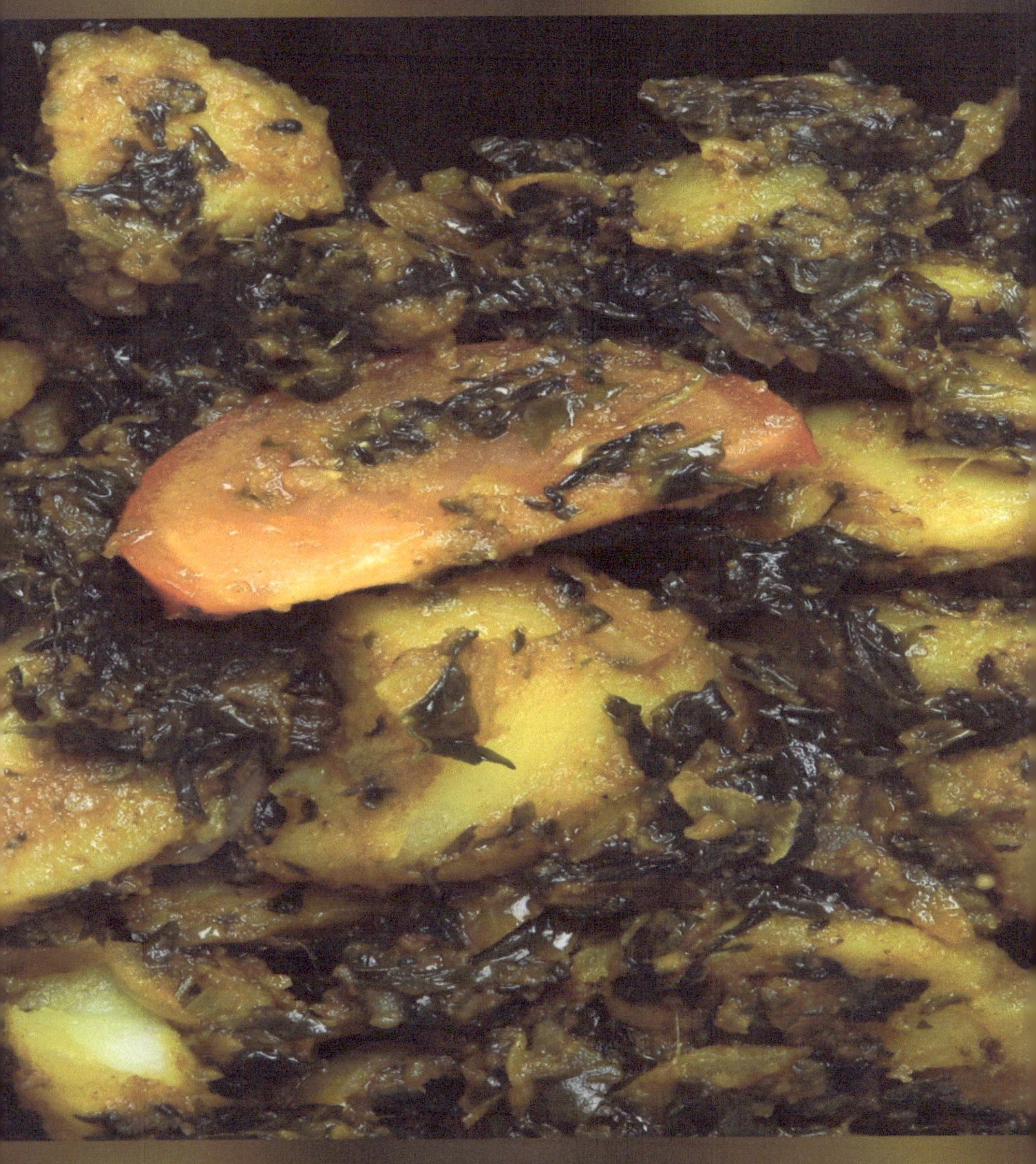

Aloo Saag
Potato and Spinach Dish

INGREDIENTS

- 3 to 4 tablespoons of ghee or sesame oil
- 3 small potatoes, diced up four ways each in wedges (boil until fork tender before cooking it with spinach)
- 1 yellow onion, chopped

- 2 tomatoes, chopped
- 2 to 3 green chilies, chopped (you can leave out if sensitive to spiciness)
- 2 spoons of garlic and ginger Paste
- ½ tablespoon ground coriander
- 1 teaspoon garam masala

- ½ teaspoon turmeric

- ½ ground cumin

- 2 tablespoons water
- 1 teaspoon brown mustard seeds
- 1 teaspoon cumin seeds
- 1 bag of frozen spinach
- 1½ teaspoons of sea salt or Himalayan salt
- ½ cup of heavy cream or as much as you think but not too much

INSTRUCTIONS

Dice 3 small potatoes four ways and boil until fork tender.

Heat 3 to 4 tablespoons of ghee or sesame oil in a large non-stick pan over medium high heat. Add the chopped onions, chopped tomatoes, chopped green chilies and spices, water, and stir. bread)

Make sure the heat is at medium.

Add the fork tender potatoes and stir in the frozen spinach, cook for a little bit or until it looks done.

Add in the heavy cream, stir occasionally and add the salt for the last bit of flavouring. Cover and simmer.

Serve with rice or roti (flat or naan.

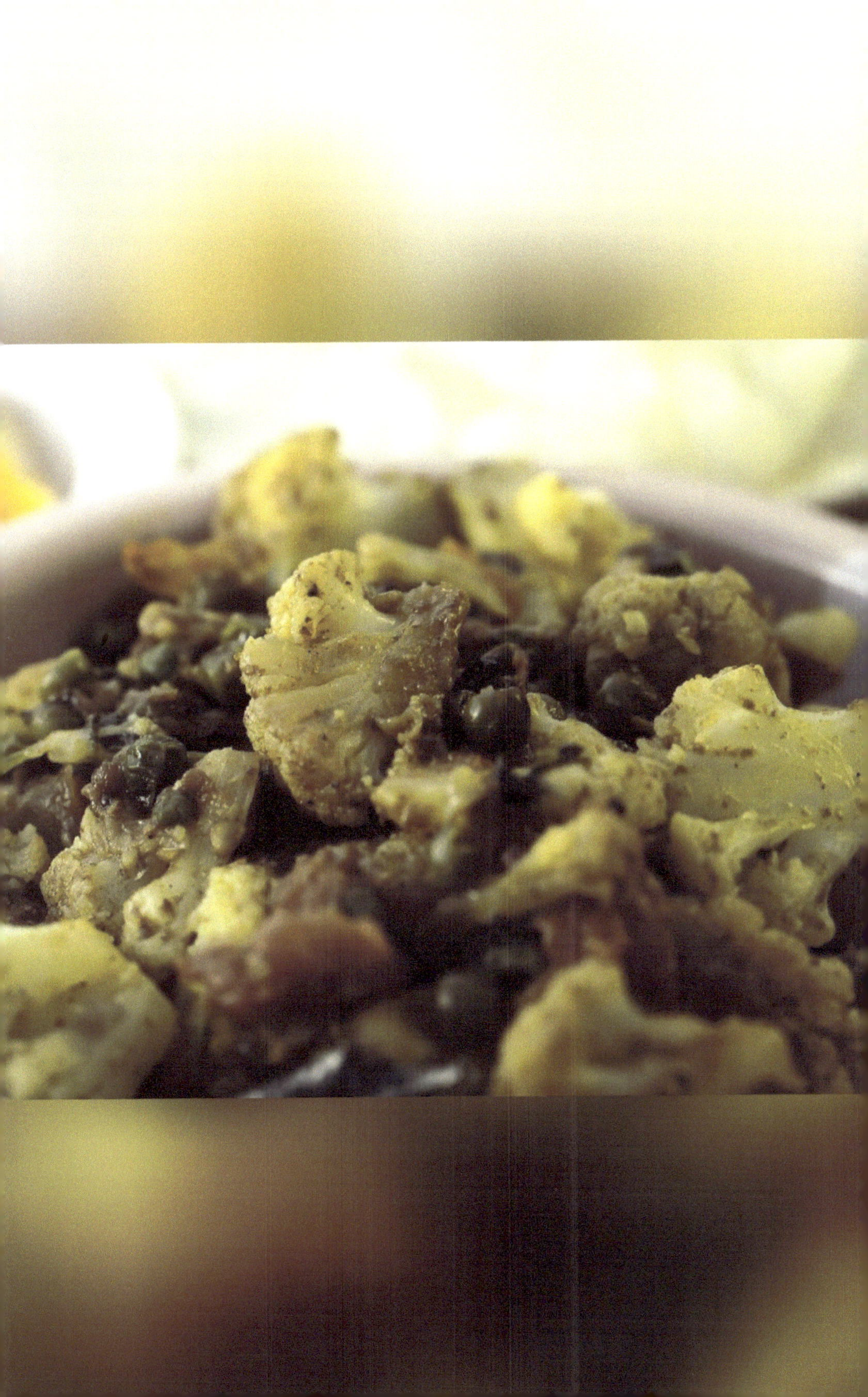

Dry Gobi Mutter
Cauliflower and Pea Curry Dish

INGREDIENTS

- 2 tablespoons oil
- 2 green chilies
- 1½ tsp ginger-garlic paste
- 1½ tsp cumin seeds
- 1½ tsp mustard seeds
- ½ tsp fenugreek seeds
- ½ tsp hing
- 1 bag of frozen cauliflower
- 1 tsp turmeric
- ½ tsp chili powder
- 1 tablespoon ground coriander
- 1½ tsp sea salt
- 2¾ cup of frozen peas
- 1 tomato, chopped
- Few dried curry leaves

INSTRUCTIONS

Heat oil over medium heat in saucepan and add cumin seeds, mustard seeds, fenugreek seeds and stir for 30 seconds. Stir in the hing.

Add chopped up chillies and garlic-ginger paste, cauliflower, turmeric, chili powder, ground coriander, sea salt and a few tablespoons of water. Coat the cauliflower by stirring. Cover and cook for 8 to 10 minutes until cauliflower is tender.

Add peas, tomato, and curry leaves. Stir and cook and cover for 5 minutes until peas are tender. Stir occasionally and add parsley. Let it stand for 5 to 10 minutes.

Serve with roti or naan.

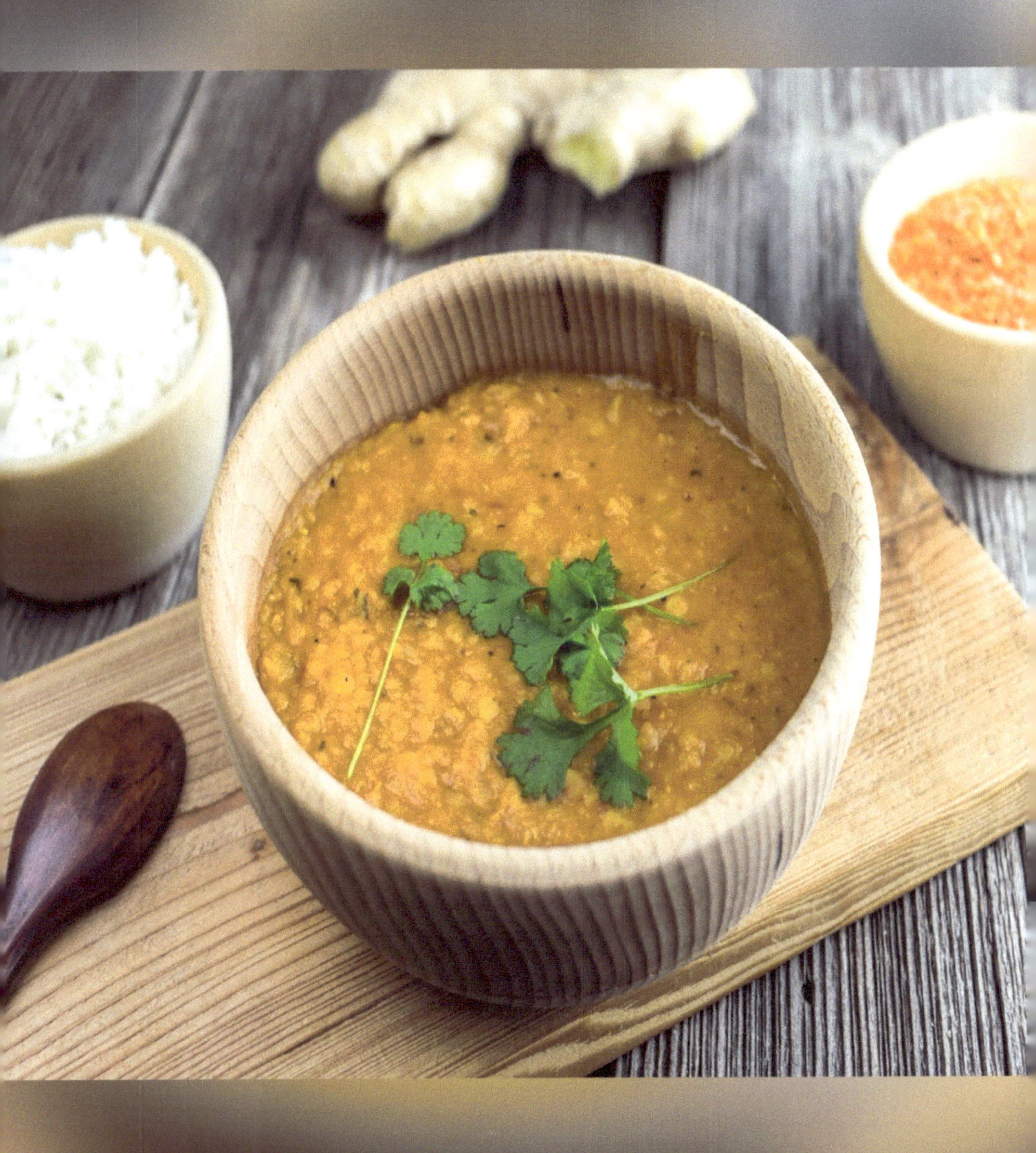

Dal Fry

Lentil Dish

INGREDIENTS

- Half cup of toor dal and half cup of masoor dal
- 2 to 2½ cups of water for Pressure cooker
- 1/3 cup chopped onions
- 1/3 cup chopped tomatoes
- 10-12 curry leaves
- ½ tsp ginger garlic paste
- ½ to ¾ tsp black mustard seeds
- 1 tsp cumin seeds
- 2 green chilies, chopped (optional)
- 1 to 2 pinches of hing
- ½ tsp garam masala
- ½ to 1 tsp lemon juice (optional)
- ½ tsp turmeric powder
- ½ tsp hing
- 1 tablespoon ground coriander

INSTRUCTIONS

Put 2 to 2½ cups of water and ¾ cup of dal with a pinch of turmeric in pressure cooker and pressure cook for an estimated 15 to 20 minutes on high. Mash up the dal a little when done pressure cooking and keep to the side.

Heat oil or ghee on high in a separate cooking pan, add mustard seed, let it cook little, add cumin and fry them, add onions and fry until it becomes transparent. Turn down to medium heat.

Add ginger-garlic paste, green chilies, curry leaves, and then stir.

Add the rest of the dried spices and chopped up tomatoes to cook, then add the mashed up dal, stir, and add a little more water as needed and salt.

Stir and simmer 4-5 minutes until smooth and slightly thick. The dal should be medium thick. Add as much water as is needed.

Serve with rice or roti or naan.

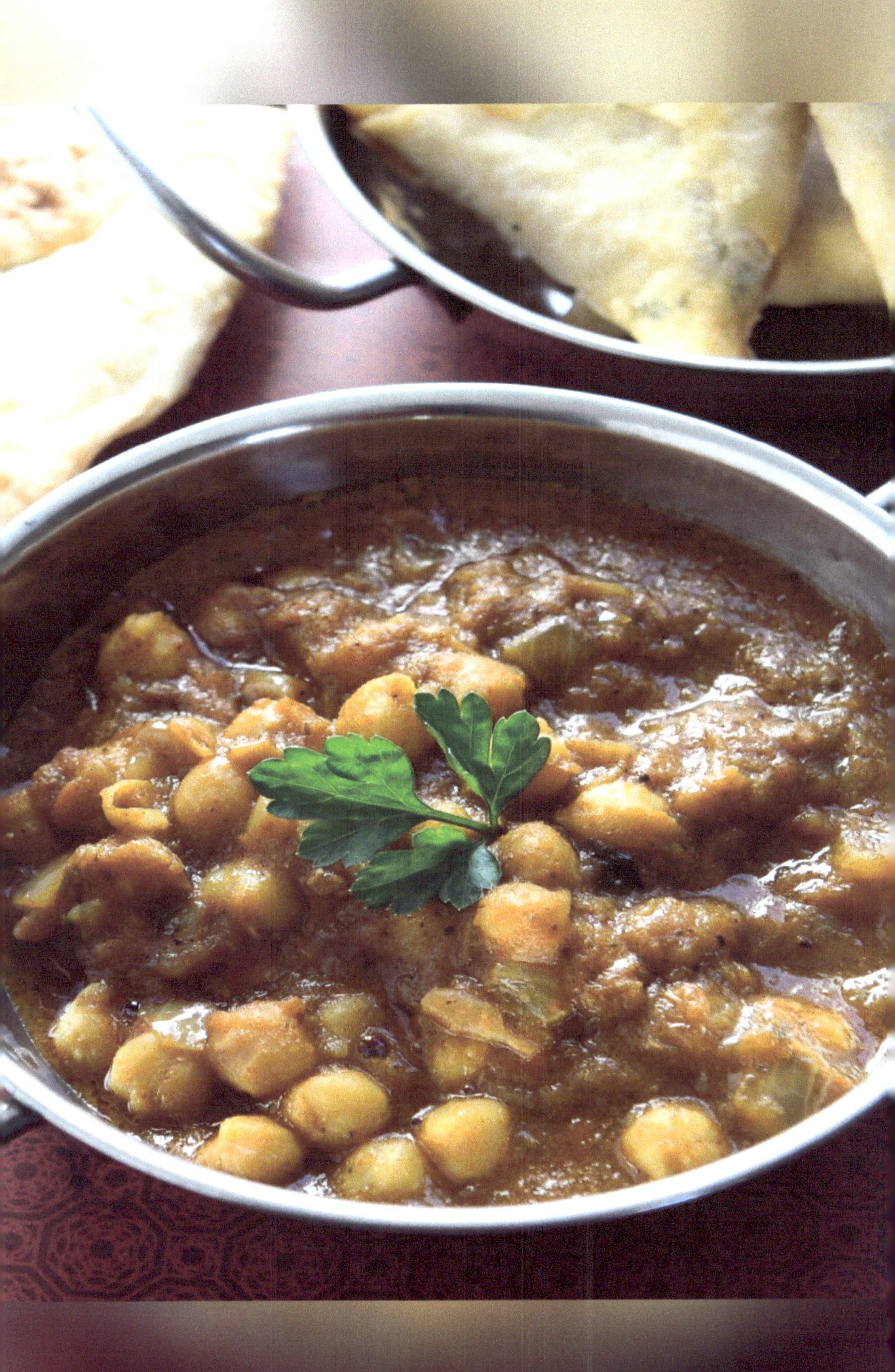

Chana Masala
Chickpea Dish

INGREDIENTS

- 1 tablespoon oil
- 1 large onion, chopped and diced
- 2 tablespoons garlic-ginger paste
- 1 tablespoon ground coriander
- 2 teaspoons ground cumin
- ½ teaspoon ground cayenne pepper
- 1 teaspoon ground turmeric
- 2 medium chopped tomatoes
- 1 cup of water
- 2 cans of chickpeas (rinse and drain them)
- 2 teaspoons cumin seeds
- 1 tablespoon mango powder
- 2 teaspoons paprika
- 1 teaspoon garam masala
- ½ teaspoon sea salt if not more
- ½ lemon juice
- 1 green chili, chopped and diced

INSTRUCTIONS

In saucepan, heat the oil, add onions, garlic-ginger paste to cook over medium heat, and then turn to medium low after 5 minutes.

Add coriander, cumin powder, cayenne, and turmeric, stir, add tomatoes and cook.

Add chickpeas and cup of water and stir

Add cumin seeds, mango powder, paprika, garam masala, salt, lemon juice, and chilies. Cover and cook for about 15 minutes or less if needed.

Serve with rice or roti or naan.

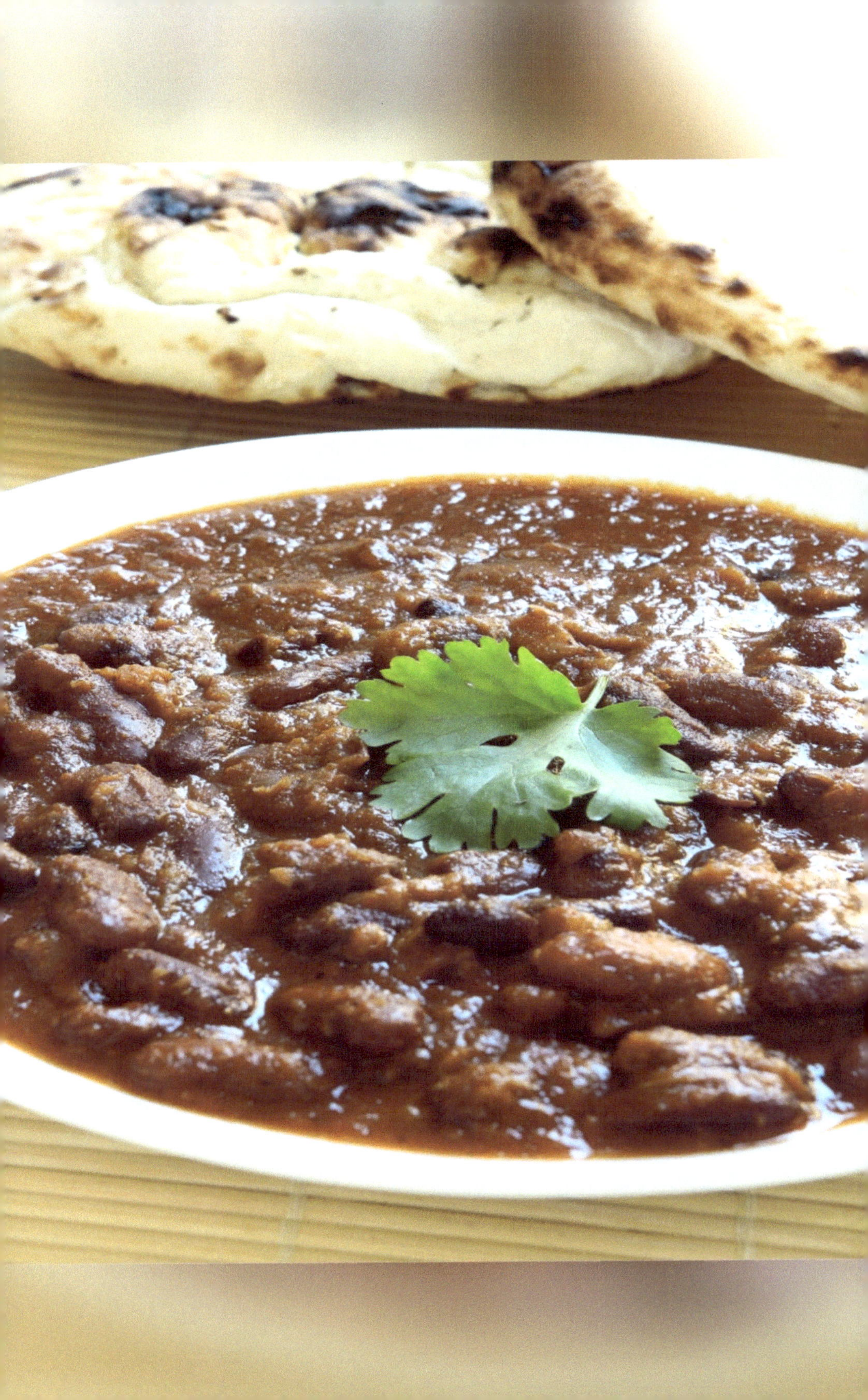

Kidney Bean Curry
Red Bean Dish

INGREDIENTS

- 4 tablespoons oil
- 1 onion, diced
- 1 green bell pepper, diced
- 2 tomatoes, diced
- 1 small can of tomato paste (need only 2 tablespoon)
- 1 teaspoon black mustard seed
- 2 teaspoons ground cumin
- 1 teaspoon split urad dal
- ½ teaspoon cumin seed
- 2 green chilies, diced
- ¼ teaspoon hing
- 1 can of kidney beans, rinsed and drained
- ¼ teaspoon garam masala
- ½ teaspoon turmeric
- 1 teaspoon curry powder
- 1 teaspoon garam masala
- Sea salt, as much as needed

INSTRUCTIONS

In the cooking pan put oil, mustard seeds, urad dal, cumin seeds, green chilies and cook on high for about 10 seconds.

Stir in the hing and onions and reduce heat to medium high and stir and cook for about 5 minutes or less.

Turn the heat down to medium and stir in green bell peppers, tomatoes and 2 tablespoons of tomato paste. Add a little water if sauce is starting to look a little dry. Cook for about 3 to 5 minutes.

Add 1 can of kidney beans after it's rinsed and drained. Add a little more water if needed. Stir and cook for 1 to 2 minutes.

Add turmeric, curry powder, garam masala and salt if needed; taste test if it's needed. Let the bean curry sit for a couple of hours, or more if needed, if you want the best taste out of it so that the flavors can have time to marinate in it.

Serve with rice or roti or naan.

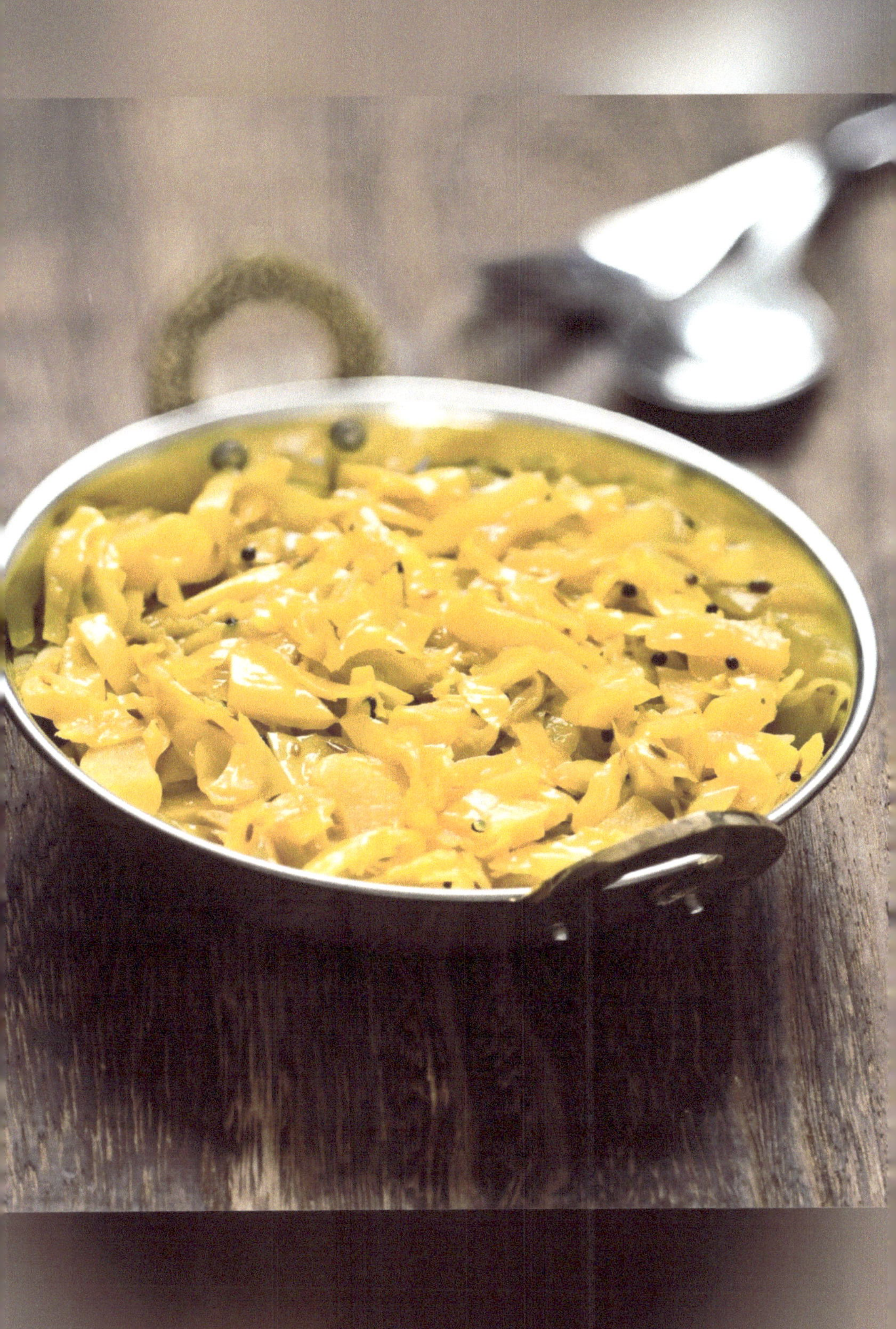

Cabbage Stir Fry
Cabbage Dish

INGREDIENTS

- 2 tbsp oil
- 1 bag of 10 oz of Angel Hair Cole Hair Cole Slaw Cabbage
- ¼ cup red onions, chopped
- ¾ tsp garlic-ginger paste
- ¼ tsp cumin
- 1 green chili, slit 4 ways
- 1 pinch of turmeric powder
- ½ tsp black mustard seeds
- 1 sprig curry leave
- Sea salt

INSTRUCTIONS

Put oil in pan on high temperature and add mustard seeds, curry leaves, slit green chilies and saute for 1 minute and then turn heat down to medium.

Add turmeric powder, onions, cumin seeds and ginger-garlic paste. Stir and cook for another minute or two.

Add the whole bag of shredded cabbage and sauté and close lid on top of the pan. Let it cook for 1 minute on medium heat throughout, remove lid and stir occasionally. When it looks cooked add as much salt as needed, then stir and fry for another 5 minutes and then turn the heat off when done frying. Avoid adding water to prevent it from going soggy.

Serve with rice or roti or naan.

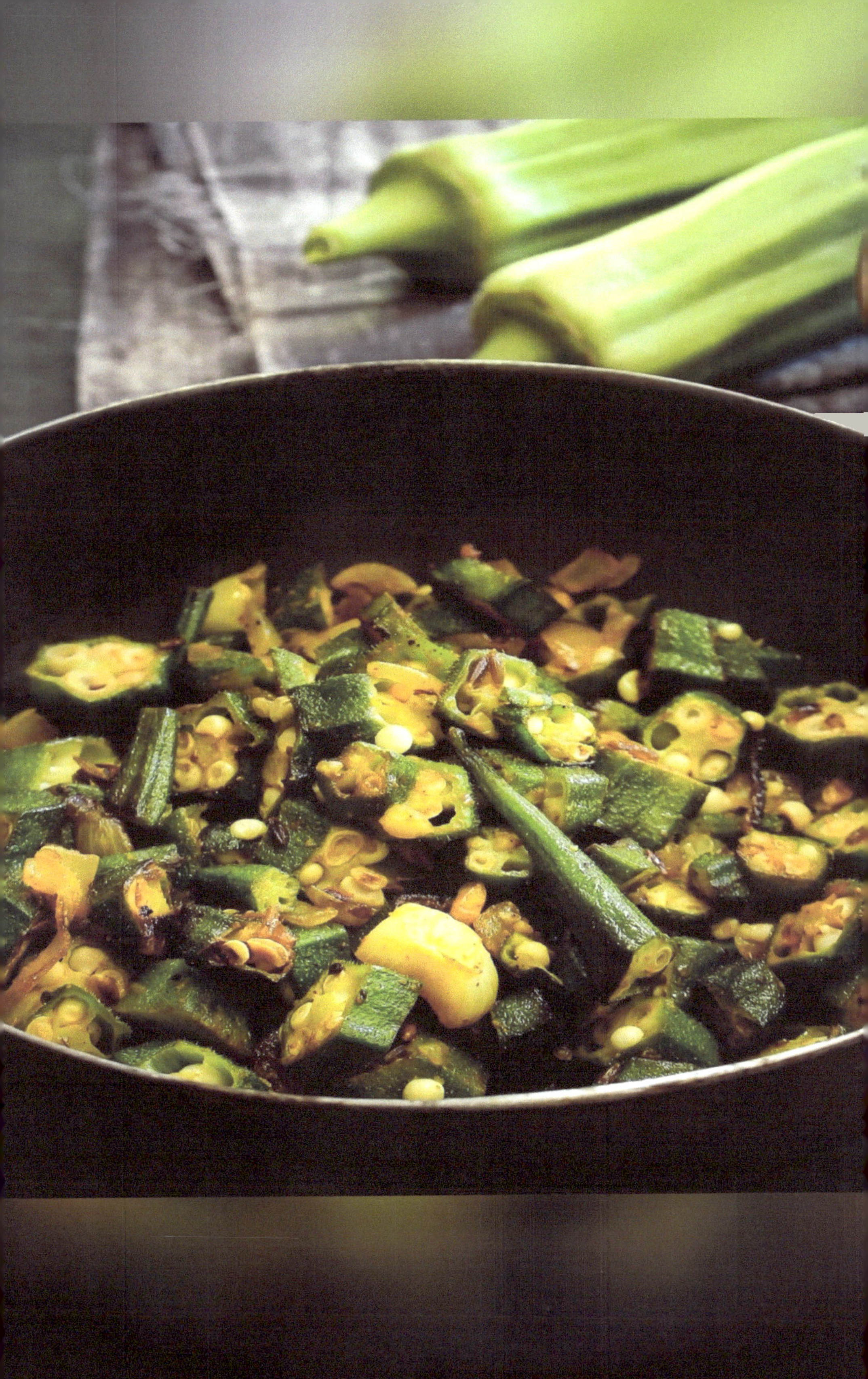

Bhindi Fry
Okra Dish

INGREDIENTS

- 2 tablespoon oil
- 1 bag of frozen okra, chopped
- 2 onions, chopped
- 1 bag of frozen okra, chopped seeds
- 1 teaspoon sambar powder

- 1 teaspoon urad dal
- 1 curry leaf
- 1 teaspoon turmeric powder
- 1 teaspoon sea salt or as much needed

INSTRUCTIONS

Turn on high heat and put oil in a pan, add urad dal, black mustard seeds, and curry leaves. Stir and cook for a minute. Then add chopped onions and put on medium heat. Cook about 2 to 3 minutes.

Add 1 can of kidney beans after it's rinsed and drained. Add a little more water if needed. Stir and cook for 1 to 2 minutes.

Add the okra, sea salt, turmeric, and sambar powder. Stir and mix. Put on low heat and let it cook for 15 to 20 minutes until it's nicely dry.

Serve with rice or roti.

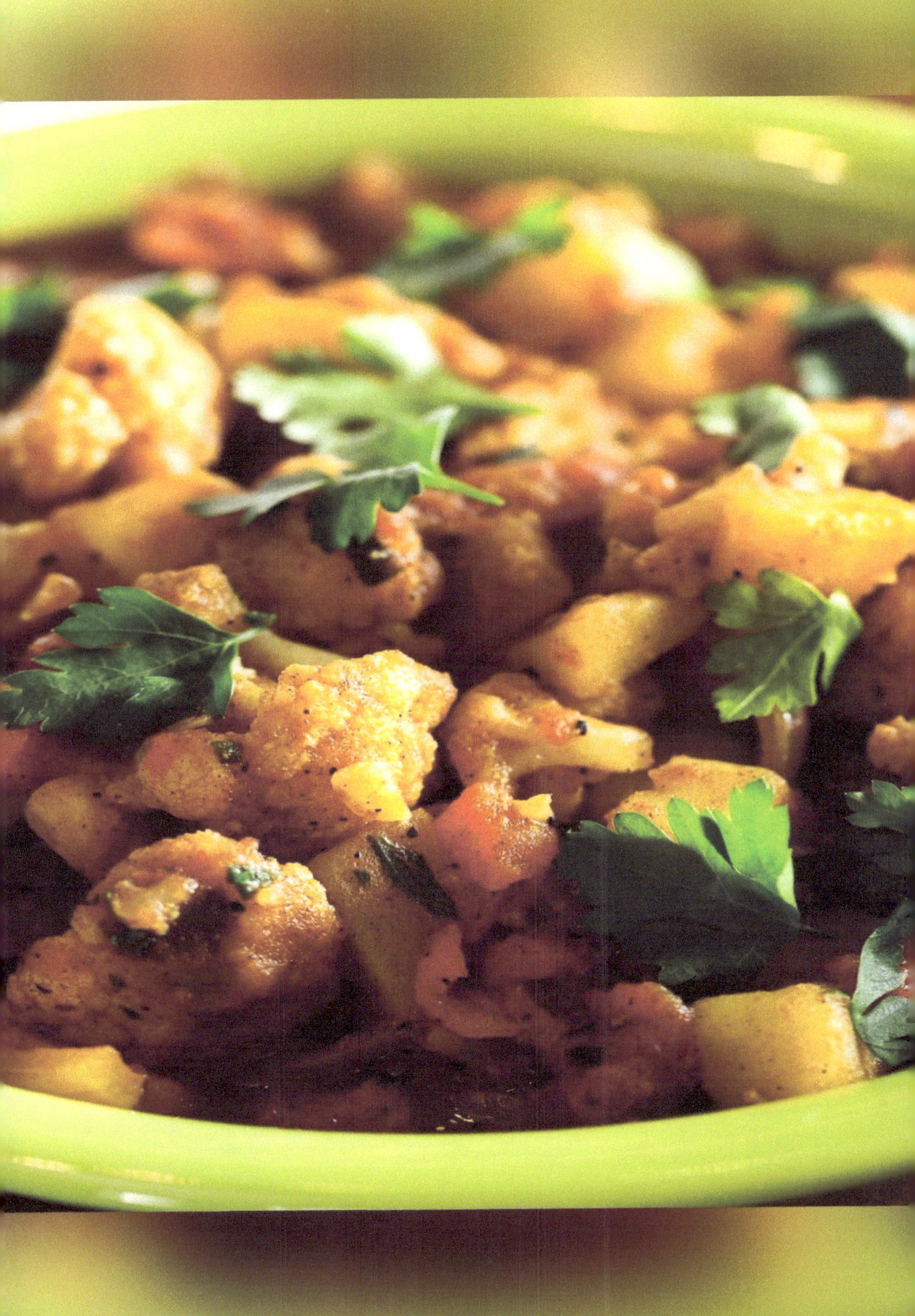

Aloo Gobi Masala
Potato and Cauliflower Curry Dish

INGREDIENTS

- 2 tablespoon oil
- 1 bag of chopped frozen Cauliflower, boiled and put in pan
- 1 tsp of ginger-garlic paste
- 2 medium Tomatoes, chopped and diced
- 2 to 3 medium Potatoes, chopped and diced into small
- pieces, boiled for 5 to 10 minutes
- ½ tsp Garam Masala
- 1½ tsp Coriander Powder
- ½ tsp Cumin Seeds
- ½ tsp of Red Chili Powder
- ¼ tsp of Turmeric Powder
- 1½ tsp sea salt
- ¼ water

INSTRUCTIONS

In a separate pot boil 1 bag of chopped frozen cauliflower for about 5 minutes with little salt, drain out water when done and keep to the side for use.

In another pot boil the chopped-up potatoes for about 5 to 10 minutes or when a little soft, drain out the water when done and keep to the side for use.

In a separate pan heat about 2 tablespoons of oil then add the chopped-up tomatoes and 1 tsp of ginger-garlic paste. Let it cook for 2 to 3 minutes and then turn heat down to medium-low where it won't burn and add all your seasonings to it; Garam Masala, Coriander Powder, Cumin Seeds, Red Chili Powder, Turmeric Powder, and Sea Salt. Cook and mix. It should look pasty. Add a little water to make it saucy looking and then add your potatoes and cauliflower in the pan and stir and cook on medium heat. Put on the lid to let the flavor infuse in and make sure you have enough water in it consistently where it won't dry up. Let it cook for 5 to 10 minutes or so and turn off.

Serve with rice.

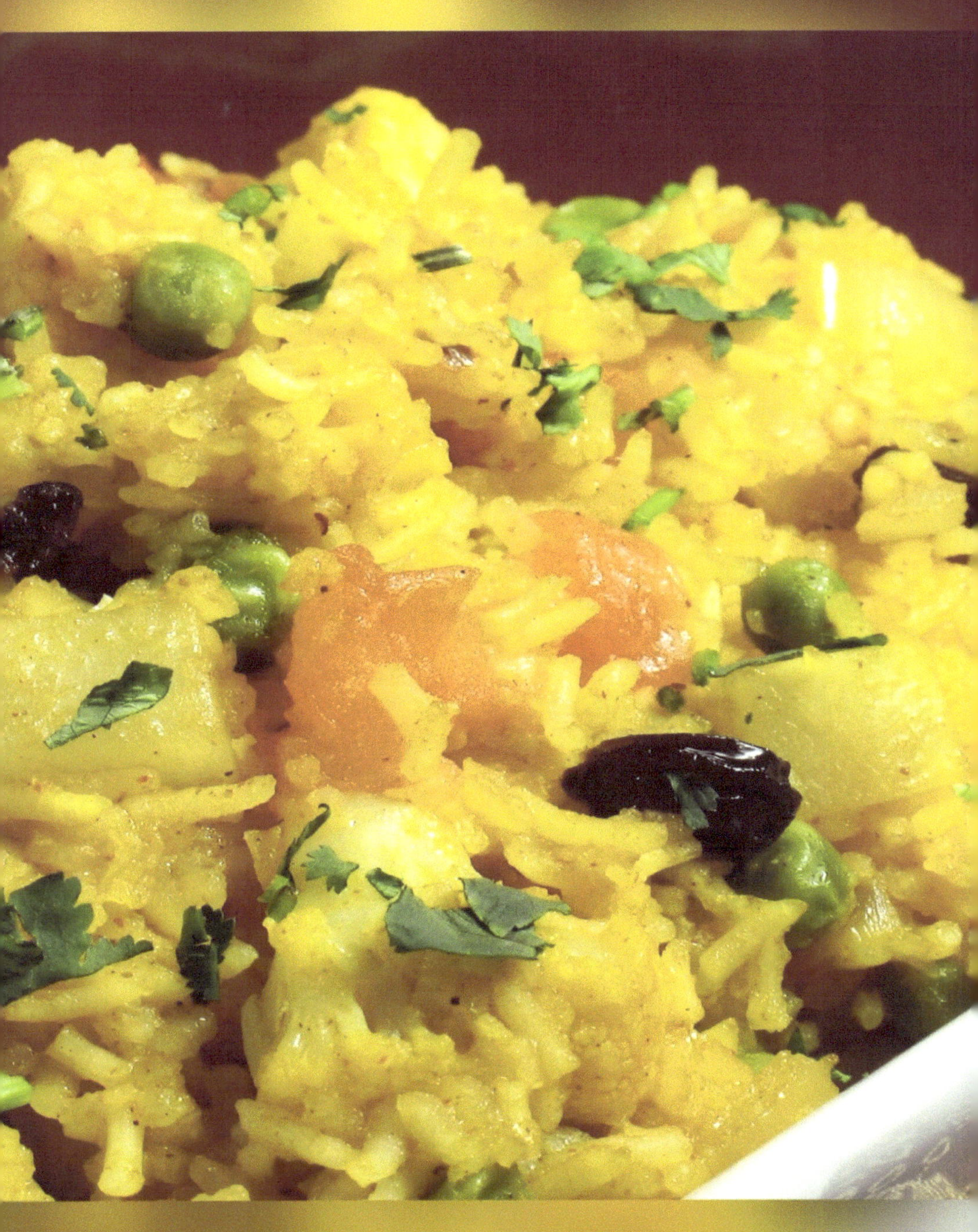

Vegetable Biryani
Vegetable Rice Dish

INGREDIENTS

- 3 tablespoons olive oil
- 1 yellow onion chopped into - ½ inch dice
- 1 tablespoon garlic minced
- 1 tablespoon ginger minced
- 1 roma tomato chopped
- ½ cup water
- ½ cup peas
- 1 carrot thinly sliced
- 2 russet potatoes peeled and Chopped
- 1 green bell pepper sliced
- 2 stalks celery thinly sliced
- 1 cup cauliflower florets
- 2 teaspoons salt
- ¼ teaspoon cayenne pepper
- ½ teaspoon black pepper
- 2 teaspoons garam masala
- 1 teaspoon coriander
- ½ teaspoon ground turmeric
- 1 teaspoon cumin
- ½ teaspoon cinnamon
- 4 cups vegetable broth
- 2 cups basmati rice rinsed and drained

INSTRUCTIONS

Add olive oil in a wok over medium-high heat.

Add the onion and cook until translucent, about 3-4 minutes.

Stir in garlic, ginger, tomatoes, and ½ cup water.

Bring to boil, and cook until the water has evaporated, about 10 minutes.

Add in the peas, carrot, potato, bell pepper, celery and cauliflower, then stir.

Add in the salt, cayenne, black pepper, garam masala, turmeric, cumin and cinnamon, and stir.

Add in the vegetable broth and bring to a boil.

Add in the basmati rice, reduce to low heat and cook (covered) for 18-20 minutes.

Turn off the heat and let sit, covered, for five minutes before you open to serve.

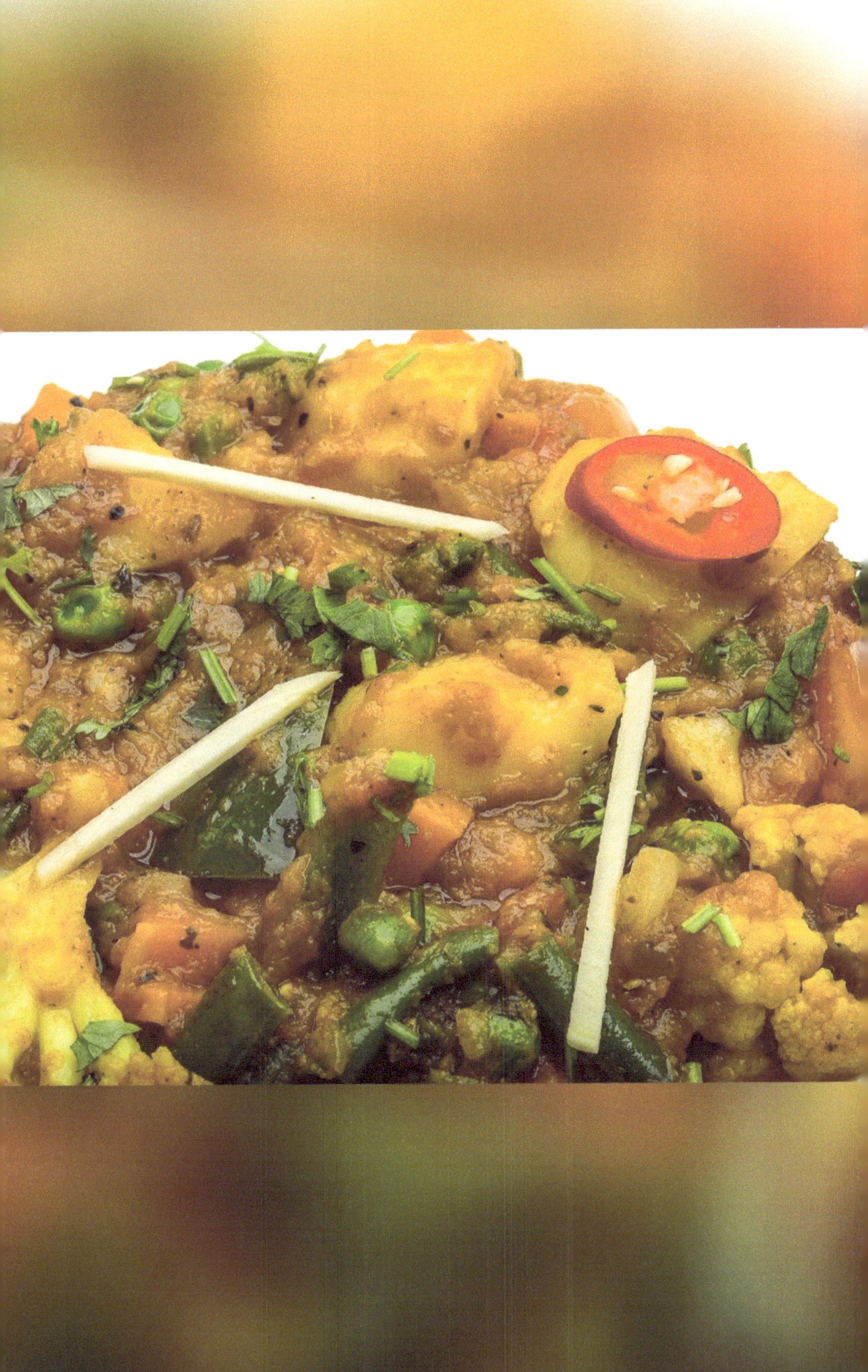

Vegetable Korma
Mixed Vegetable Dish

INGREDIENTS FOR THE BASE

- half of medium onion, sliced
- 1 tbsp ginger/ garlic paste
- 1 single Serrano pepper, sliced
- 1/4 cup raw cashews
- 1 hand full of cauliflower florets (from frozen bag is fine)
- 1/2 cup water

INSTRUCTIONS FOR THE KORMA

- 1 tbsp oil
- 2 small tomatoes, diced
- 1 medium potato, peeled and diced
- 2 cups frozen mixed vegetables
- 2 tbsp curry powder
- 1 tsp ground turmeric
- 1 tsp garam masala
- ½ tsp cinnamon
- ½ tsp coriander powder
- ⅛ tsp ground cardamom
- 1½ tsp brown sugar
- ½ tsp black pepper
- Salt, to your liking
- ½ cup coconut milk
- 3/4 cup plain yogurt

INSTRUCTIONS

- Take all of your above ingredients and put in a blender or processor and blend until it turns into paste.

- Set to the side.

INSTRUCTIONS

- In a large flat pan add your 1 tbsp oil, heat the pain on high.
- Add your base/paste from your blender into your pan. Turn heat down to medium.
- Add your potatoes and all your spices, stir and cook. Add your diced tomatoes and vegetables.
- Turn heat to medium high.
- Add your yogurt and coconut milk last and stir and cook and turn heat back down to medium after a few minutes of cooking. Put a lid on to let the food cook in its seasonings and flavors. Once the potatoes are tender, turn your heat off.
- It should take about 20 to 25 minutes to cook. You can taste the flavors best once the Korma cools down and the spices have had time to settle in the food.

INDEX OF TERMS

Saag: Spinach
Aloo: Potato
Chapati: Roti (flat bread)
Chai: Tea
Ghee: Clarified Butter
Asafetida Powder: Hing Seasoning
Haldi: Turmeric Seasoning
Lal Mirch Powder: Red Chili Powder
Hari Mirch: Green Chili
Kali Mirch: Black Pepper
Kasuri Methi (Kasoori Methi): Dry Fenugreek Leaves
Methi Ke Dane: Fenugreek Seeds
Jeera: Cumin Seeds
Rai: Black Mustard Seeds
Adrak: Ginger

Lahsun: Garlic
Bhindi: ladyfingers, Okra
Chane: Chickpeas
Dhania Powder: Coriander Powder
Sabut Dhania: Coriander Seeds
Amchur Powder: Dry Mango Powder
Namak: Salt
Kari Patta (Kadipatta): Curry Leaves
Mutter: Peas
Dal: Lentils
Phul Gobhi (Gobi): Cauliflower
Band Gobhi: Cabbage
Sabzi: Vegetable
Tamatar: Tomato
Piaz: Onion

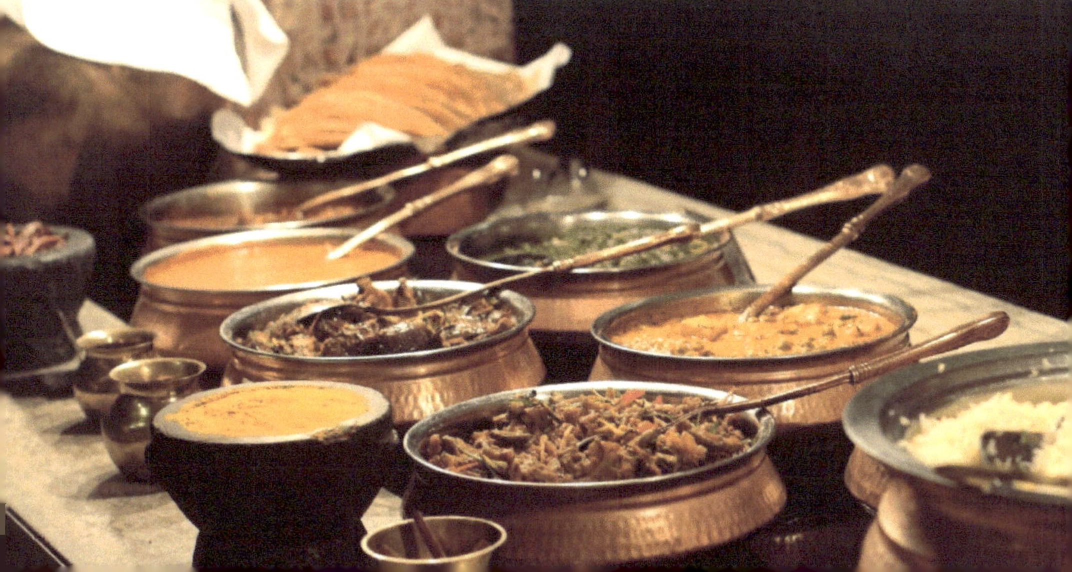